Top Favorite Asthma Natural Treatments

"Discover The Best Asthma Remedies To Reduce Attacks"

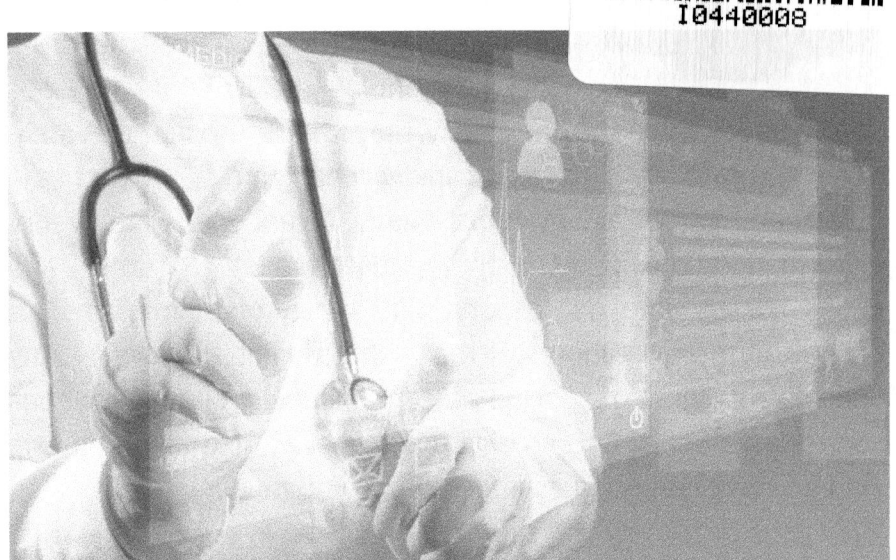

Rudy Silva Silva, Natural Nutritionist

Cures With Asthma Treatment Remedies © 2011, updated 2018 by Rudy S. Silva

Printed in the United States of America

Table of Contents

Chapter 1: Introduction

In this e-book, you will find an explanation of what asthma is and what is being used to treat it. In later chapters, I give you some natural remedies that have historically worked to reducing or even eliminating, in some cases, asthma.

My philosophy on health is that you use natural remedies first when you know you have a specific condition you want to eliminate or to get relief from. If the natural remedies don't work and the condition is getting worse, then it time to see your doctor.

In cases of severe asthma, it is best to get control of it by going to the doctor to get medication. And, even after your doctor prescribes drugs, you can continue to inform yourself, test, and use natural remedies. Care must be taken if you are using drugs since some herbs interact with them causing unacceptable side effects.

Asthma is a widespread persistent inflammatory condition of the lung airways whose cause is not totally understood. It's a disorder of the respiratory system in which the passage of air to the lungs sporadically narrow causing coughing, wheezing, and shortness of breath which often worsens at night. This tightening is typically short-term and reversible, but in severe attacks, asthma can result in death.

The term Asthma most frequently refers to bronchial asthma, another inflammation of the airways, but it is also used to refer to cardiac asthma, which develops when fluid builds up in the lungs as a complication of heart failure.

Asthma is caused by the inflammation of the airways where air flows into and out of the lungs. The muscles of the bronchial tree become taut and the lining of the air passages to enlarge, which reduces airflow and produces the characteristic asthmatic wheezing sound.

An asthma attack can also occur as an allergic reaction to an allergen or other substance (acute asthma), or as a part of a complex disease cycle, which includes reactions to stress or exercise (chronic asthma).

Alternate Names For Asthma Include Bronchial Asthma, Exercise-Induced Asthma - Bronchial, Reactive Airways Disease (RAD)

Chronic Asthma

In chronic asthma, inflammation can be accompanied by irreparable airflow limitation. In pre-school children underlying pathology may not exhibit considerable bronchial hyperreactivity, and there is also no evidence chronic inflammation is a basis for the episodic wheezing which is associated with viral infections.

Chapter 2: Characteristic Features of Chronic Asthma

Having said that however long-term follow-up in these developing countries suggests asthma problems may become more frequent as the population becomes more 'westernized'.

Studies of occupational asthma suggest a high proportion of the workforce, perhaps up to 20%, may become asthmatic if exposed to potent sensitizers.

Asthma has three characteristics:

- airflow limitation
- airway hyperresponsiveness
- Inflammation of the bronchi with its associated plasma exudation, edema, and smooth muscle hypertrophy, mucus plugging, and epithelial damage.

Asthma can be divided into:
- **Extrinsic** - implying a definite external cause
- **Intrinsic** - when no causative means can be identified.

Extrinsic asthma

This occurs most regularly in individuals who show a positive skin-prick reaction to universal inhalant allergens. Positive skin-prick tests to these inhalant allergens are shown in 90% of children with persistent asthma, yet only 50% of adults tend towards this trend.

Intrinsic asthma

This usually starts in middle age, though many sufferers with adult-onset asthma show positive skin tests and on closer questioning often give a history of respiratory symptoms, which are compatible with childhood asthma. Asthma Attacks

Chapter 3: Causes Of Asthma

Asthma attacks are caused by airway hyper receptiveness. The most common causes of an asthma attack are very small lightweight particles transported through the air and inhaled into the lungs.

When they enter the airways, these particles, which are known as environmental triggers, cause an inflammatory reaction in the airway walls, which results in an asthma attack.

Allergens

For some people environmental triggers are allergens. These are natural substances, such as plant pollen and mold spores, animal dander (tiny pieces of animal hair and skin), undigested food, and fecal material from dust mites and cockroaches.

Allergens, which the body sees as a foreign substance, activate a response from the immune system. A specific antibody immunoglobulin E, IgE, combines with the allergen. This combination, IgE and allergen, attach themselves to a specialized white blood cell called "mast cells". This attachment then triggers the release of histamine, which causes swelling and inflammation.

These same allergens usually cause little or no response in non-allergic people.

The allergens involved in asthma are similar to those

in rhinitis, a histamine reaction that occurs in the throat, eyes, and nose when airborne particle irritate those areas.

The particle size of pollens (>20 microns) means they are more likely to cause conjunctivitis, rhinitis, and pharyngitis as well as asthma. Allergens from fecal particles of the house-dust mite are the most important extrinsic cause of asthma worldwide.

Chemical Irritants

Chemical irritants trigger an inflammatory response differently to allergen-triggered asthma.

Some people are sensitive to common chemical irritants, such as perfume, hairspray, makeup, and household cleaners.

Other chemical irritants include industrial chemicals and plastics, as well as many forms of air pollution, such as exposure to high levels of ozone, car exhaust, wood smoke, and sulfur dioxide.

Physiological Triggers

Aggravation from within the body is known as physiological triggers and includes exercise and infections, such as the common cold. Sometimes eating certain types of food can cause an asthma attack.

Chemicals found in food or drugs such as aspirin and ibuprofen can be especially problematic for many asthma sufferers. Emotions, such as expressions of grief, shouting causes and triggers of asthma

Environmental Pollution

Epidemics

Major epidemics of asthma have been recorded when large amounts of allergens have been released into the air, (e.g. there was a soybean epidemic in Barcelona.)

Further insignificant epidemics of asthma have occurred during periods of heavy atmospheric contamination in industrialized areas, which is caused by the presence of high concentrations of sulfur dioxide, ozone, and nitrogen dioxide in the air.

Food

There are certain foods that can trigger an asthma attack, such as artificial colors (like yellow food dye 5), monosodium glutamate, cheese, sauerkraut, alcoholic beverages, vinegar, benzoic acid or sodium benzoate (a preservative), mushrooms, soy sauce, bread with yeast

Salicylate, found in aspirin, or foods that contain it sometimes can trigger an asthma attack. Sulfites, used on dried fruits, can also be an asthma trigger.

When you have allergies to foods most likely, you have a deficiency in a digestive enzyme and this prevents you from digesting or breaking down this food into its simple chemical form. The result is these undigested particles can get into your blood and cause an allergic or asthma attack.

Emotion

Asthma is also influenced by certain emotions such as laughing, crying, anger, panic, etc. But many in the medical community believe there is no proof people with asthma are any more psychologically disturbed than their non-asthmatic peers. However, it is not possible to have an illness without it having an emotional or trauma component associated with it. Our brain and body is not a split organism where our brain and body work independently of each other.

Having asthma is most likely related to birth traumas where the newborn is being suffocated by the birth process. This trauma causes weakening the lungs and the bronchioles. And if the child has or had parents that were overprotective or dominating, this could further imprint the birth trauma of suffocation.

And, there are many other scenarios that could weaken a person's lungs and bronchioles during childhood. You might know what yours were.

In his book, How to Get Well, 1974, Paavo Airola, Ph.D., says,

"Extensive studies show that there are two basic causes of asthma: one, the typical allergic reaction to one or more allergens; two, psychic factors. Doctors agree that many young asthmatics (according to studies, about 25%) have in common a 'deep-seated emotional insecurity and an intense need for parental love and protection'. When emotional causes are suspected, these must be dealt with before biological and nutritional treatments can be effective."

Emotions and feelings, such as apprehension, concern, anxiety, and panic can cause muscular tension and contraction around the bronchioles. Over a long time, these tensions can cause muscle spasms and weakening of the bronchioles, which can then lead to asthma as an adult.

In his book, Cleanse & Purify Thyself, 1998, Richard Anderson, N.D., N.M.D., says,

"Our own research indicates that Love is the great key. When we understand that Love is the natural state of our beings and when Love is not flowing through our beings every moment, then some other emotion or concept is interfering. These interferences are usually emotions of great intensity or some quirk in our point of view, such as the habit of judging conditions, things, or people in negative ways, and most of the time they are unconscious. One of the activities we all need to initiate is to remove these conscious and unconscious negative emotions so that Love may flow through us. Here in lies one of the most important point in this book."

Hypoglycemic

If you are hypoglycemic, high sugar levels in your blood can trigger an asthma attack. What happens is when your sugar blood level gets too high, your pancreas overacts or malfunctions with high levels of insulin rapidly bringing down your sugar to a low level.

Low levels of sugar in your blood because you're liver to release an excess of sugar into your blood to even out the low blood sugar levels. Then, more insulin is released to get the excess liver sugar down again.

These reactions of the pancreas and liver, in trying to control the blood sugar level, force the lungs to act up to help these organs fight off invaders – lungs interprets high insulin levels to indicate the presence of pathogens in the blood – so the lungs release histamine. This histamine causes blood to rush to the bronchioles, which can result in inflammation and spasms. These spasms can result in an asthma attack.

When the pancreas is malfunctioning and the adrenal gland is weak or not functioning properly, the adrenals will not be able to release enough cortisone to counteract the lung's release of histamine.

What causes the high blood sugar levels in the first place?

High blood sugar levels are caused by the foods you eat. Eating foods that are high on the glycemic index such as white flour products, processed foods, sugar, sodas, and sweet bread all lead to high sugar in the blood.

Acid Body

An acid body is one that contains too much acid in the blood and in the lymph liquid. This results in lowering the pH of those liquids making them more acidic than they should be.

The normal body is alkaline. This means that the pH of various body liquids and organs have a normal pH and this is what is required to minimize disease and have good health.

An acid body means that too much acid is being released into the body as a result of acid activities:

Eating too much meat at mealtime

Eating too much processed and packaged foods

Not eating enough raw fruits and vegetables

Drinking too many sugary drinks

Mixing and eating too many different foods at mealtime

Over-exercising

Leading a worrisome and stressful life

Having an angry, vindictive, or negative personality

In Felicia Drury Kliment's book The Acid Alkaline Balance Diet, she points out,

"That acidic waste (in the form of gas) is a factor in all asthmatic lung problems is confirmed by the discovery of Dr. Benjamin Glaston, associate professor of pediatric pulmonary medicine at the University of Virginia. According to Dr. Glaston, an asthmatic's breath is 1,000 times more acidic than normal breath. Normal breath is slightly alkaline with a pH of 7.4, but when asthmatics are sick and wheezing, their breath pH drops to 5.0 – into the acidic range of the pH scale. That asthma sufferers have acidic breath is not surprising, given that acidosis, a blood pH that is below the normal alkaline pH, has long been associated with asthma. It's possible that just the presence of toxic acidic gas in the lungs can bring on an asthmatic attack."

Look for what kind of diet is needed to keep your body alkaline – listed in the natural remedy section to follow.

Toxic Colon

A toxic colon can lead to many diseases. When the colon is not cleansed yearly, toxins can build up and create acid gas. This gas can penetrate the colon walls move into the blood and travel into the kidneys and into the lungs.

This acid waste, in lungs, can create mucus and irritate the lining of the lungs triggering a histamine release. This release can cause bronchiole spasms, which in turn can result in an asthma attack.

Keeping the colon free of constipation is necessary for minimizing the acid gas from forming and escaping into the lungs.

In my ebook on "How to reduce or eliminate constipation using 77 natural remedies", I give a complete look at what is constipation, how to eliminate it using natural remedies and how to prevent it by eating the right kinds of foods.

Chapter 4: Asthma Symptoms

Non-steroid anti-inflammatory drugs (NSAIDs). NSAIDs, chiefly aspirin, have a major role in the development and precipitation of attacks in approximately 5% of people with asthma.

Immediate asthma

This is the most common response. An attack begins within minutes of contact with the allergen, reaches its maximum in 15-20 minutes and subsides after 1 hour.

Late-phase reactions

Following an instantaneous reaction, many asthmatics may develop more prolonged and sustained attacks that respond inadequately to the inhalation of bronchodilator drugs.

Dual asthmatic response

This is a combination of an early reaction followed by a late reaction.

Recurrent asthmatic reactions

Development of a late-phase response is associated with increases in the underlying level of airway hyperreactivity that individuals can show with systematic episodes of asthma on subsequent days.

Asthma Symptoms & Signs
Clinical features

People experiencing asthma exhibit symptoms virtually identical to those suffering from airflow limitation, which is caused by COPD. (Chronic Obstructive Airways Disease). The symptoms for both are usually worse during the night.

Wheezing attacks and shortness of breath are more or less universal in both conditions. A cough is a frequent symptom that will often predominate, and can often be misdiagnosed as another respiratory disorder.

There are many variations in the regularity and duration of asthmatic attacks. Some individuals have only one or two attacks a year lasting a few hours, whilst others may have attacks lasting for weeks.

Unfortunately, asthma is a major cause of impaired quality of life. It has an impact on work as well as recreational and physical activities and emotions.

Symptoms of Asthma

Wheezing which usually begins suddenly is episodic may be worse at night or in the early morning. It can be aggravated by exposure to cold air, by exercise, and by heartburn and it.

Resolves spontaneously is relieved by bronchodilators

Other Symptoms include

- cough with or without sputum (phlegm) production
- shortness of breath which is aggravated by exercise
- breathing requiring increased work
- intercostals retractions (pulling of the skin between the ribs when breathing)

Emergency Symptoms of Asthma

- acute difficulty in breathing
- bluish color to lips and face
- severe apprehension
- fast pulse
- sweating decreased level of consciousness (severe drowsiness or confusion) during asthma attack death

Additional symptoms associated with asthma

- nasal flaring
- chest pain
- tightness in the chest

An abnormal breathing pattern, in which exhalation (breathing out) takes more than twice as long as inspiration (breathing in) breathing which temporarily stops coughing up bloodChapter 5: Asthma Diagnosis & Tests

Physicians typically diagnose asthma by looking for characteristic symptoms such as intermittent problems with breathing, which can include wheezing, coughing, and shortness of breath. When these symptoms alone fail to establish a diagnosis of asthma, doctors will usually use spirometry testing.

Trigger Identification

Identifying a specific trigger of a person's asthma is frequently more difficult than an initial diagnosis. An asthma sufferer might develop an asthma attack when using a particular cosmetic or household cleaning product. So when triggers are difficult to identify, a series of allergy skin tests are useful to determine what they are.

Correct Diagnosis

Making a correct diagnosis is tremendously important because if asthma is correctly diagnosed it can be treated more appropriately.

A diagnosis of asthma involves all of the following:

A detailed history, which would include:

A family history of asthma, allergies, hay fever, and eczema; children will have a greater chance of developing the above if there is a family history of allergies and asthma.

A child's medical history including:

When parents first noticed the child developed breathing problems; history of nasal stuffiness (rhinitis), itchy eyes (allergic conjunctivitis) and eczema, which are common accompaniments to asthma, and hives (urticaria).

A history of a recurrent and persistent cough following a cold, frequent cold, croup, seasonal changes (i.e. worse in the spring and autumn), exercise limited by breathing problems, waking at night with symptoms. school absences, emergency room visits (hospitalizations)environmental history

Physical examination: i.e. listening to the lungs with a stethoscope; examination of nasal passages etc.

Chest x-ray to exclude the likelihood of breathing problems being caused by something other than asthma.

Blood tests and sputum studies.

Allergy prick skin testing: Skin tests can confirm a presence or absence of allergies, but they must be correlated with the history of symptoms shown.

Spirometry If testing children who are less than five years old, this test is not commonly indicated because a certain amount of effort and cooperation is required. However, it's a very good trustworthy method of making an asthma diagnosis. Any difficult or troublesome asthma should be confirmed objectively by performing a spirometry test.

Challenge tests: Exercise challenge tests and methacholine inhalation tests are procedures, which are used most frequently in clinical laboratories to assess airway responsiveness.

Differential diagnosis: Other possible causes of shortness of breath, wheeze, and cough plus chest tightness need to be investigated in order to rule them out. These can include such illnesses as heart disease, other lung conditions, and gastro-oesophageal reflux.

A trial use of asthma medications: If asthma medications are taken and an improvement in symptoms is seen this further supports a diagnosis of asthma.

Tests may include:

Peak expiratory flow charts

Exercise tests

Histamine or methacholine bronchial provocation test

A trial of corticosteroids

Blood and sputum tests

Chest X-ray

Skin tests

Allergen provocation tests

Peak expiratory flow charts

Measurements of PEFR on waking, prior to taking a bronchodilator medication and before bed after a bronchodilator, are very useful in demonstrating the variable airflow limitations characterizing asthma.

It's also useful in the longer-term evaluation of the sufferer's disease and its response to proffered treatment. Peak flows should always be measured over several days and preferably over a weekend or short holiday if the effect of the asthma sufferer's work exposure is also being studied.

Exercise tests

These are widely used in the diagnosis of asthma in children. Ideally, the child should run for 6 minutes on a treadmill at a workload, which is sufficient to increase their heart rate above 160 beats per minute. Alternative methods use cold air challenge.

Histamine

This test indicates the presence of airway hyper responsiveness, which is a feature found in most asthmatics. It can be predominantly useful in investigating those people whose main symptom is a cough.

Trial of corticosteroids

All asthma sufferers presenting with a severe airflow restriction should undergo formal trials of steroids. Prednisolone 30 mg orally is usually given daily for 2 weeks with their lung function measured before and immediately after the course.

A significant improvement confirms the benefits of this type of treatment for the asthma sufferer. If the trial is for 2 weeks or less, the oral steroids can be withdrawn without tailing off the dose, and should be replaced by inhaled corticosteroids in those people who have responded and are thought will benefit from this medication.

Blood and sputum tests

Individuals with asthma often have an increase in the number of eosinophils in the peripheral blood. However, the presence of large numbers of eosinophils in the sputum is a more useful diagnostic tool.

Chest X-ray

This has slightly limited use as there are no diagnostic features of asthma on a chest X-ray, although during an acute occurrence or in chronic severe disease over inflation is a characteristic often found in a chest x-ray.

Skin test

Skin-prick tests should be performed in all cases of asthma to help identify allergic triggers.

Chapter 6: Asthma Treatment

Although there is no cure for asthma, effective management is available for preventing attacks and controlling and ending attacks soon after they have begun.

Asthma medications are taken orally or inhaled in vapor form using a metered-dose inhaler. This is a hand-held pump, which delivers medicine directly to a person's airways.

There are two kinds of asthma medication: bronchodilators, which reduce broncho-spasms; and anti-inflammatory medications, which reduce airway inflammation.

Immunotherapy is another treatment option for asthma caused by allergens. This form of therapy modifies a person's allergic response by repeated exposure to small amounts of allergens.

By breathing into a PEFR, a small hand-held device called a flow meter, an asthmatic can find out when their airways are first starting to narrow. When the PEFR falls, asthma medication is probably needed to prevent an attack.

Note:

PEFR and medication should only ever be used under a physician's.   guidance.
There are two basic kinds of medication for the treatment of asthma:

Long-term control medications – These are used on a regular basis to prevent attacks and not to be used for treatment during an attack.

These include:

Inhaled steroids (e.g., Azmacort, Vanceril, AeroBid, Flovent) prevent inflammation leukotriene inhibitors (e.g., Singulair, Accolate) long-acting bronchodilators (e.g., formoterol, Serevent) help open airways cromolyn sodium (Intal) or nedocromil sodium aminophylline or theophylline (This isn't used as frequently as it was in the past) a combination of anti-inflammatory and bronchodilators, using either separate inhalers or a single inhaler (Advair Diskus)

Quick-relief (rescue) medications – which are used to relieve the symptoms during an acute attack. short-acting bronchodilators (e.g., Proventil, Ventolin, Xopenex, and others) oral or intravenous corticosteroids (e.g., prednisone, methylprednisolone), which help to stabilize severe episodes of asthma.

People with mild asthma (infrequent attacks) can use their relief medication as needed, but those with persistent asthma problems should take their control medications on a regular basis to prevent their symptoms from occurring.

A severe asthma attack requires a medical evaluation and may even require hospitalization with oxygen, intravenous therapy and medications being required.

How to Approach Asthma Management

A winning approach to asthma management is critically dependent on using the correct anti-inflammatory medications with bronchodilators, **which** are needed for immediate and occasional relief of symptoms of asthma.

Anti-Inflammatory - Preventers: Anti-inflammatory medication is used to treat the inflammation caused by exposure to inducers.

Bronchodilators - Relievers (Rescue medication) Bronchodilators are used to relieve Broncho-constriction, which is provoked by triggers.

Medications: Anti-inflammatory

A successful move towards decent asthma management, both in and out of an acute hospital setting is dependent upon the accurate use of anti-inflammatory treatment and bronchodilators being prescribed for immediate and occasional relief of any symptoms shown.

Anti-inflammatory medications work mostly by interfering with the activity and chemistry of immune cells, such as mast cells, which cause inflammation in the airway walls. Anti-inflammatory medication also helps rest the airway muscles that narrow and constrict during broncho-spasms.

Anti-Inflammatory Medications (Preventers)

These: prevent and reduce inflammation, swelling and mucus in the airways put a stop to symptoms such as a cough, wheeze, and breathlessness need to be taken on a regular basis are slow acting (over hours or weeks)

Types of Anti-Inflammatory Drugs

There are steroidal and non-steroidal anti-inflammatory drugs.

The most common ones include:

A-Steroids

beclomethasone (Beclovent®, Vanceril®, Becloforte®)

budesonide (Pulmicort®)

flunisolide (Bronalide®)

fluticasone (Flovent®)

B-Non-Steroidal

sodium cromoglycate (Intal®)

nedocromil (Tilade®)

Corticosteroid Inhalers

Corticosteroid drugs are the most effective Preventers. They work by reducing and preventing airway inflammation, swelling and mucus.

They must be used regularly and **do not** have an instant effect. This means they have **no value** whatsoever if an effect is needed right away.

Corticosteroids inhalers are less toxic than oral corticosteroids like prednisone. But, because of their side effects, Disodium cromoglycate or Cromolyn is a better choice as an inhaler.

The Side effects of Corticosteroid Inhalers
There are few side effects at low doses

High doses might cause growth suppression; studies have shown children whose asthma is not controlled don't grow as quickly as other children. hoarseness, dryness of the throat and mouth.

Sore throat

Overgrowth of Candida albicans yeast in the mouth called thrush, which can be prevented by rinsing the mouth and gargling. Using a holding chamber can also help prevent side effects.

Corticosteroids should not be used long term. They are useful for short-term to gain control over asthma.

Alert: Corticosteroids suppresses the immune system and should not be used when you have any sort of infection. Overuse can result in side effects similar to the oral corticosteroids.

Corticosteroid Tablets

Corticosteroid tablets or Prednisone®:

These are used when inflammation becomes severe. They reduce inflammation, swelling & mucus, and help bronchodilators work better. They start to work within a few hours, but may take several days to have a full effect. They are often used for short periods of time just to get the inflammation under control.

There are lots of side effects if used on a long-term basis such as water retention, bruising, puffy face, increased appetite, weight gain, and stomach irritation.

Other Preventers

Other preventers are Intal® and Tilade®. They are non-steroidal and again used to reduce inflammation. Disodium cromoglycate also known as Cromolyn is a synthetic derivative of khellin, a natural compound. Khellin was derived from the Ammi visnaga plant and used by ancient Egyptians to treat asthma and angina.

Cromolyn or Disodium cromoglycate has activity similar to quercetin, a bioflavonoid. It works by stopping the release of histamine and other compounds from mast cells. It is used to prevent allergic reactions but will not stop them once they are underway.

Disodium cromoglycate (Intal®) most effective in preventing asthma attacks triggered by exercise for mild asthma this can protect against the effects of cold air it requires 4-6 weeks to be effective it has few side effects.

Disodium cromoglycate is well tolerated by the body and has few side effects. Despite the aerosol not tasting good, it is tolerated quite well by the body. Side effects occur in a few people and when they do they experience bronchospasm, coughing, wheezing, joint pain hives, skin rash or nausea. I rare side effect is a severe allergic reaction.

Ketotifen (Zaditen®)

Ketotifen is used for mild asthma, and it can be useful for asthmatics who also suffer from hay fever. It helps to reverse inflammation of the airways, it can be used orally and comes in tablets or syrup, but requires regular use of 8-12 weeks to become effective. Its side effects include drowsiness and weight gain.

Bronchodilator Medications (Relievers)

Bronchodilators are the most extensively used medications for controlling unexpected asthma attacks and for preventing attacks brought on by physical activity or exercise. Theophylline is a bronchodilator that works by relaxing the muscles surrounding the airways.

These:

Are rescue medications, therefore are used only when needed, and rarely on a regular basis (unless the asthma is under inadequate control)

- Provide quick relief of symptoms shown
- Relax the muscles of the airways
- Are useful with exercise-induced bronchospasm
- Are usually in blue devices

Types of Bronchodilator Drugs

The most common bronchodilators are:

B$_2$-Agonists – come in inhaler or pills, but inhaler most frequently used because of fewer side effects Anticholinergic Inhaler, Theophylline

B$_2$-Agonists

salbutamol (Ventolin®, Apo-Salvent®, Novo Salmol®) fenoterol (Berotec®)terbutaline (Bricanyl®) pirbuterol (Maxair®)

B2-Agonists are rescue medications which:

Relax the muscles around the airways, which allows the breathing to become much easier within minutes. The effectiveness of use lasts 3-6 hours.

Are used only when needed and rarely on a regular basis, unless the asthma is under inadequate control.

Make the airway muscle less likely to contract.
Are usually in blue devices.

When to use B2 – Agonists

To relieve symptoms of a cough, chest tightness, wheezing and shortness of breath a few minutes before exercising or before exposure to any trigger known that might worsen asthma

Side effects of B2-Agonists include:

- trembling
- nervousness
- flushing
- increased heart rate
- increased dependence on attacks
- increase blood pressure
- insomnia and anxiety
- headache, dizziness
- nausea
- heart palpitations

Anticholinergic Inhaler
Atrovent®

Atrovent opens the airways by blocking signals from the nervous system, which cause the airways to become contracted. It takes one to two hours to reach its maximum effect; therefore, it shouldn't be used as an immediate emergency medication.

Side effects

There are few side effects; a bad taste is probably the only one.

- Theophylline
- TheoDur®

- Uniphyll®
- Phyllocontin®
- TheoLair®

Theophylline is an oral bronchodilator, which works directly to relax the airway muscle.

It can be used at night-time if shortness of breath disturbs sleep or more frequently if the asthma condition is very severe. Theophylline levels can be affected by other medications – so it's important the physician is aware of all medications asthmatics are taking, including over-the-counter drugs.

Side effects include:

- Diarrhea
- Nausea
- Heartburn
- Loss of appetite
- Headaches
- Nervousness, insomnia
- Rapid heartbeat
- Upset stomach
- Increase urination

Use of theophylline will always result in side effects. Children who use theophylline will have even more severe side effects.

Theophylline is a toxic chemical that has a very small margin of safety. The required dose is close to the toxic level and this drug requires close monitoring by a doctor. Typically this drug might be used for acute asthma attacks.

Theophylline is not now commonly used in the treatment of asthma.

The drugs that have theophylline are :

- Bronkodyl
- Elixophyllin
- Slo-bid
- Theobid
- Theo-Dur
- Somophyllin_T
- Uniphyl

Medications: Inhalation Devices

Asthma medications come in many forms

- Metered Dose Inhaler (puffer)
- Dry Powder Inhalers (Diskhaler®, Turbuhaler®)
- Nebulizer

Chapter 7: Using A Metered Dose Inhaler Correctly

Metered Dose Inhalers (MDI)

Metered dose inhalers, MDI, or puffers, deliver an exact dose of medication to the airways when used correctly. Unfortunately, many asthma sufferers don't use MDI's correctly and don't receive the correct dosage. Therefore if the asthma sufferer can't use a puffer, a holding chamber may be needed.

One advantage of using an MDI is it is very portable. remove the cap from the mouthpiece and shake the inhaler breathe out to the end of a normal breath position the mouthpiece end of the inhaler about 2-3 finger widths from your mouth open your mouth widely and tilt your head back slightly or alternatively close your lips around the mouthpiece start to breathe in slowly, then depress the container once continue breathing in slowly until the lungs are full once you have breathed in fully, HOLD your breath for 10 seconds or as long as you can if you need a second puff, wait one minute and repeat the steps

Taking Care of a Metered Dose Inhaler

- Keep the inhaler clean.
- Wash the mouthpiece
- Check the expiry date.
- Check to see how much medication is in the inhaler.

Holding Chambers

Holding chambers are devices with one-way valves, which hold the medication for a few seconds after it has been released from the puffer. They used by people who:

Have trouble coordinating the hand-breath step
Are using high-dose steroids.

Using a holding chamber can prevent

A hoarse voice

A sore throat.

Care of the holding chamber

Whichever holding chamber is used, it must be cleaned at least once a week with warm water and air-dried.

Dry Powder Inhalers

General points include:

The medicine is only inhaled when a breath is taken.
The devices do not contain propellants to help the medication go into the lungs.

The devices are portable and come in convenient sizes.

Proper Use of a Diskhaler®

To load the Diskhaler®, remove the cover and cartridge unit Place a disk on the wheel with the numbers facing up and slide the unit back into the Diskhaler® Smoothly push the cartridge in and out until the number 8 appears in the window, the Diskhaler® is now ready for use. Lift the lid up as far as it will go - this will pierce the blister Shut the lid

Take breaths in and out

Place the mouthpiece between your teeth & lips - make sure you don't cover the air holes at the sides of the mouthpiece and tilt your head back slightly

Breathe in deeply & vigorously

Hold your breath for 10 seconds or as long as you can, sometimes 2 or 3 forceful breaths in are needed to make sure all the medication is taken.

If a second blister is prescribed, advance the cartridge to the next number & repeat the steps

Care of Diskhaler

Any remaining powder must be cleared to ensure proper dosage.

Proper Use of a Turbuhaler®

Unscrew the cover and remove it

Holding the device upright, turn the colored wheel one way & back the other until it clicks - it is now loaded Breath out. Place the mouthpiece between your lips and tilt your head back slightly breathe in deeply and forcefully hold your breath for 10 seconds or as long as you can if a second click is prescribed, repeat the steps

Care of Turbuhaler

Keep the Turbuhaler clean.

Nebulizers (Compressors)

A nebulizer or compressor is used chiefly for small children and elderly people. Each treatment requires sitting quietly for 20-30 minutes whilst the drug is nebulized from a liquid to a mist.

Care of Nebulizer and Equipment

Wash the mask with hot, soapy water. Rinse well and allow it to air dry before re-use
.

Here is one cautious word on inhalers. Felicia Drury Kliment, an alternative researcher, and writer, in her book The Acid Alkaline Balance Diet, gives us this report on inhalers,"Those asthma patients who rely most heavily on inhalers, however, run twice the risk of dying. Two studies conducted in New Zealand and Canada documented the dangers of bronchodilators. These statistics became real to me when a friend of mine, Jacob, died from the overuse of an inhaler.

Jacob pulled the inhaler out of his pocket whenever he wheezed. One day he had a full-scale asthmatic attack. He used the inhaler, but it didn't open up his breathing passages. He had used it so often that it has lost its effectiveness. With no one around to rush him to a hospital he died."

In a later chapter, I list a variety of natural remedies that you can try so that you can lessen your dependence bronchodilators.

Chapter 8: Management of Asthma

Asthma is very common and causes substantial morbidity. The aims of treatment are: to abolish the symptoms to re-establish normal or best possible long-term airway function to decrease the risk of severe attacks to facilitate normal growth occurring in children to reduce absence from school or employment.

This involves:

Patient and family instruction about asthma patient and family input in treatment prevention of identified causes where the possible use of the lowest effective doses of convenient medications to minimize short-term and long-term side-effects.

Control of extrinsic factors

Measures should be taken to avoid contributing allergens such as the house-dust mite, pets, molds, and certain foodstuffs, particularly in childhood.

Evasion of house-dust mites is now achievable with efficient and secure covers for bedding and changes to people's living accommodation. Smoking should be avoided at all cost.

Other agents (e.g. preservatives and coloring materials such as tartrazine) should be avoided if shown to be a causative factor. Fifty percent of those sensitized to work-related agents could be cured if they are kept permanently away from contact.

This emphasizes:

The significance of rapid identification of extrinsic causes of asthma and their removal wherever possible (e.g. occupational agents, family pets) Once extrinsic asthma is started, it can become self-perpetuating.

How to manage catastrophic sudden severe (brittle) asthma

This is an unusual variation of asthma in which patients are in danger of sudden death despite their asthma being well controlled between attacks. Severe life-threatening attacks can occur within hours or even minutes.

Brittle Asthmatics should ensure they have

emergency supplies of medications at home, in the car and at work oxygen and resuscitation kit at home and at work nebulized β_2 agonists at home and at work self-injectable epinephrine (adrenaline): two Epipens of 0.3 mg epinephrine at home, at work and to be carried by the asthmatic at all times prednisolone 60 mg Medic Alert bracelet.

Asthma Prevention

Avoiding known allergens and respiratory irritants can significantly reduce asthma symptoms. If somebody with asthma is responsive to dust mites, contact can be reduced by encasing mattresses and pillows in allergen-impermeable covers, removing carpets from bedrooms, and by vacuuming regularly. Exposure to dust mites and mold can be reduced by lowering indoor humidity.

If an individual is allergic to an animal that cannot be removed from the home, the animal should be kept out of that person's bedroom and off furniture.

Filtering material can be placed over the heating outlets to trap animal dander. Exposure to cigarette smoke, air pollution, industrial dust, and irritating fumes should also be avoided as much as possible.

Allergy desensitization can be helpful in reducing asthma symptoms and medication use, but the size of the advantage compared to other treatments is not known.

Asthmatics can also prevent and control attacks by limiting their exposure to environmental triggers.

Carpets, beddings etc should be regularly cleaned.

A mask should be worn

Bathe pets regularly but avoid using shampoo all of the time – it's the saliva and dandruff, not hair that can cause an attack.

Steer clear of pollutants and irritants

Cyclic allergies to pollen and mold spores can be reduced by avoiding the outside during peak periods of activity

Asthma Complications

- Respiratory fatigue
- Pneumothorax
- Side effects of any medication used
- Death

Asthma Prognosis (Prospect)

There is no cure for asthma, though symptoms sometimes decrease over a period of time. With appropriate self-management and therapeutic treatment, most people with asthma can lead normal lives.

Although asthma often improves in children as they reach their teens, it is now realized the illness frequently returns in the second, third and fourth decades of life.

Previously data indicating a natural reduction in asthma through adolescent years has led to childhood asthma being treated as an intermittent disorder. However, it is now considered that airway inflammation is present continuously from an early age and frequently persists even if the symptoms resolve.

Furthermore, airways remodeling accelerates the process of decline in lung function over a period of time. This has led to a review of the management strategy for asthma, encouraging the early use of efficient and effective controller drugs and environmental measures from the time asthma is first diagnosed.

In the following chapters, you will find some natural remedies that have proven successful in helping people with their asthma. Use those remedies that you feel comfortable and safe with. Remedies and especially some herbal formulas work slower than drugs, but they are more balanced and can help to rebuild those tissues that are weak and in need of repair.

In a book by Michael Castleman, Blended Medicine, 2000, says,

"Mainstream M.D.'s also prescribed anti-inflammatories and bronchodilators – drugs that open narrowed bronchial tubes – to help control asthma symptoms. 'In my experience, these medications help, but they're not the answer,' says Richard Firshein, D.O. assistant professor of family medicine at the New York College of Osteopathic Medicine. 'In managing my own asthma, I've had tremendous success with a comprehensive program that includes drugs as well as alternative approaches. The same goes for my patients. Within 6 weeks of beginning treatment, 95 percent of them are able to cut back on their medications. About 60 percent reduce their dosages by half.' "

Of course, you should never stop taking any asthma medication or change your dosage without your doctor's okay."

Chapter 9: Natural Remedies For Asthma Relief

It is important to get a doctor's diagnosis on whether you have asthma or not. If you do have asthma, then using drugs to get relief when you have a severe or life-threatening attack becomes a necessity.

Once you are set with the correct doctor's prescriptions, then you owe it to yourself to start looking for natural remedies that can work with your existing drugs and to eventually replace them. Using drugs for asthma simply suppresses the symptoms, suppresses your immune system, creates minor and major side effects and does nothing to eliminate or cure your asthmatic condition.

What drugs will do for you is give you temporary relief and with long-term use make you dependent on them and in some cases create the condition you are trying to eliminate. They also will give you side effects that can be more dangerous than the asthma you have. Drugs are good for short-term use so that you can have the time to find a natural and safer way to deal with your asthma.

Natural Asthma Remedies

In this chapter, I list a variety of different natural asthma remedies that you can experiment with. Some remedies will work better for you than for another person. Each person is different and needs a different nutritional or nutrient to help reduce, eliminate or even cure an asthmatic condition.

Care must be taken as you use these remedies. Start with a small dose to see the results and then increase the dose as you see improvements. You can check with your doctor to see if there can be any interference with any drug that you are using.

The remedies are not listed in order of importance but are listed in alphabetical order so you can find them easier.

Antioxidants

Antioxidants are critical to take for asthma. Weakness in the bronchial tubes and lungs leads to sensitivity to various outdoor pollution and internal food particles. The various sources of chemicals you eat and particles in your breath can be free radicals that attack your internal wall linings making them weak. This weakness can lead to spasms, mucus accumulation, and inflammation.

Take antioxidants to neutralize free radicals, reducing the number that can attack and damage the and interior of your body and lungs. This keeps your body strong and able to react and protect itself when undesirable chemicals enter your body.

You can take a supplement, which contains many antioxidants. Look for a product that is called "antioxidant formula."

This formula should contain selenium, vitamin A, C, E. Other antioxidants are alpha lipoic acid, glutathione, and quercetin. Most fruits have bioflavonoids, which are antioxidants.

Balsam of Peru Resin

Balsam of Peru is a resin from a tree in El Salvador. From a 20-year-old tree, they remove the resin and create an oil that has a vanilla-like fragrance.

This oil has been used for skin diseases, wound healing, coughs, lung ailments, asthma, and colds. It has antibacterial, antiseptic and anti-parasitic properties.

Use 5 drops in water 2 times per day. Here's where you can get it.

Balsam of Peru at this Website, scan down the page to find it.

Black Mocha Coffee

Black mocha coffee has been found to relax the bronchial tubes and prevent their constriction for up to 6 hours. This coffee is a preventative remedy for asthma and should be used a couple of hours before it is needed. In addition, it can provide relief during an attack. Use up to 2 cups if you weigh up to 125 lbs.

Continual use of this coffee for asthma will lessen its effect and should only be used when really needed. In fact, when continually used, asthma attacks will become more severe, so use this remedy in emergencies.

Black mocha coffee has been found to have a methylated xanthine, which is related to theophylline that has been made into a drug.

If you are taking theophylline or a similar drug, do not use coffee because of possible side effects.

Proper Breathing

Most people who have anxiety, are worrying, upset, or stressed tend to take shallow breaths. This keeps their feelings pushed down and keeps them from dealing with uncomfortable personal situations. When you have asthma, this type of breathing can start an asthma attack. By learning to breathe right and maintaining this type of breathing most of the times, you can minimize an asthma response.

In his book, Blended Medicine, Mr. Castleman, describes how to develop proper breathing,

"Dr. Firshein recommends regular practice of a technique called belly breathing. 'Most people think that breathing is automatic.' He notes, 'Few know that there's a right and wrong way to do it. Bell breathing helps to condition the lungs and diaphragm to prevent asthma attacks.'

To try belly breathing, lie on your back and place a book on your abdomen. As you inhale and exhale, your abdomen should expand and contract enough to move the book up and down several inches.   Practice this exercise for 5 minutes three to four times a day."

Cranberries

Cranberries are good for stop asthmatic wheezing. Here's what to do:

Put cranberries in a juicer. Add some warm distilled water to the juice to dilute it.   Drink a cup of this and add a teaspoon of honey, if you like. Experiment to see how much you need to drink to stop your wheezing.

Digestive Enzymes

Using digestive enzymes when you have asthma is a good idea. Digestive enzymes help reduce inflammation, fibrin, and clean the blood of foreign particles. These enzyme activities strengthen your immune system and give it more power to work on the allergens that may trigger an asthma attack.

Use two to three digestive enzymes capsules before or during a meal to digest your food properly.   For asthma, take two to three capsules between meals so the enzymes can get into your blood and digest any foreign matter in your blood that can cause allergies or an asthma attack.

Bromelain

Bromelain is a digestive enzyme that is found in pineapple. It's capable of reducing inflammation and swelling and for this reason has been used for asthma

Bromelain also activates a chemical that promotes the breakdown of fibrin. Fibrin is a chemical that repairs open wounds, internal wounds, and weak tissue by creating fibrin deposits. If you are over 35, fibrin is not balanced with your body's enzymes. This results in excess fibrin deposits at inflamed locations, eventually causing more sickness and disease.

To balance and control excess fibrin activity, you need to take digestive or systemic enzymes. Systemic enzymes are enzymes that work throughout the body to attack blood impurities and dissolve fibrin.

As a supplement take 500-750 mg a day. You can also add fresh pineapple to your diet since it is high in fiber and other nutrients.

Digestive and Systemic Enzymes

Digestive enzymes are used to help you digest your food and improve your food assimilation. They reduce stress on your gastrointestinal walls, help maintain your body's pH, detoxify your body, and replace your pancreatic enzymes.

Digestive enzymes help to reduce the allergens that might get into your blood. When your food is not properly digested. Undigested food reaching intestines can be absorbed into your blood. These undigested particles are allergens to your body and activate your body to release antibodies and histamine. This, in turn, creates allergic symptoms that can cause asthma attacks.

Undigested food that reaches the colon eventually leads to constipation. Constipation can create toxins that eventually get into your blood making your blood toxic.

Toxic blood can be routed to the lungs to be excreted when the liver, kidney, and colon are overworked with toxins.

Use digestive enzymes when you are hypoglycemic since your pancreas can be weak and not putting out enough digestive juices to digest your food properly in the small intestine.

Take a good digestive enzyme that you can get at health food stores. Take 2 capsules with each meal or read the label for guidance.

Systemic enzymes help reduce mucus accumulation, swelling, and inflammation. They improve circulation and speed the healing of tissue, stimulate the immune system, breakdown mucus so it flows easier, strengthen the body and improves your overall health.

One important fact about systemic enzymes is they eliminate fibrin, which is at the center of most inflammatory conditions and illness.

Systemic enzymes are found deep in your body. They are in your tissues, organs, and cells where they help in all types of chemical reactions that your body is involved in.

Both digestive and systemic enzymes are available in capsules, so you can easily supplement your diet.

Take systemic enzymes between meals, because it allows them to reach the small intestine and get absorbed into the bloodstream where they can do their work.

Some systemic enzymes are enteric enzymes, which mean they are coated so they will not dissolve in the stomach. This allows them to move into the small intestine where they will be absorbed into your bloodstream.

The systemic enzyme, Vitalzyme, contains serrapeptase that is mixed with other nutrients and enzymes. Just put Vitalzyme or serrapeptase into the Google engine. This will bring in a flood of sites for you to choose a good systemic enzyme.

Start by taking three systemic enzymes between meals for a total of 9 per day. Then increase this to 3 the following week. Then you can increase the amount every week until you see results in your reaction to allergens or asthma triggers. You cannot overdose taking a lot of systemic enzymes.

If you are troubled with stomach or any other internal ulcer, do not use digestive or systemic enzymes, since they will aggravate your ulcer. There is a product put out by Tyler, which is called GS Simalase which is designed for people with ulcers. You can find this product on the Internet.

Eucalyptus Leaves

Eucalyptus leaves have a long history of being effective in relieving symptoms of asthma. These leaves can be used to drink as a tea. As an essential oil, you can use it to inhale, from a face steamer. In a face steamer or other distilled water steamer, place a couple of drops of eucalyptus oil and inhale the fumes for a few minutes.

Eucalyptus leaves help to reduce that mucus that accumulates in the bronchia's that hamper breathing.

Do this in the evening just before bedtime or when you feel the need to.

Essential Oils

Breathing the fumes of essential oils is an excellent way to get quick relief from asthma. When first starting to use essential oils and a hot distilled water diffuser, approach the vapors slowly so that you know that the fumes will not irritate you and cause an asthma attack.

Mix the following essential oils into a brown dropper bottle.

- 5 parts eucalyptus
- two parts lavender
- two parts myrrh
- three parts chamomlle

Do not use essential oils for internal use. Use only a brown dropper glass bottle to hold your essential oils. These oils tend to dissolve plastic bottles and are affected by the light.

Here are an asthma and bronchitis remedy that is recommended in Jeanne Rose's book, The Aromatherapy Book, 1992,

"For bronchitis and asthma keep a small bottle of [cedar] oil mixed about half and half with Eucalyptus [then add] Chamomile"

The formula is:

- 2 oz water
- 10 drops Cedar oil
- 10 drops Eucalyptus oil
- 2 drops Chamomile oil

"You should Inhale whenever necessary. You can also use it on a hanky that you can inhale discreetly whenever necessary to reduce asthmatic symptoms."

You can also add a couple of drops of cedar oil and eucalyptus oil into a diffuser and inhale the fumes.

Do not use cedar oil if you have high blood pressure or heart problems.

Another essential oil called **Ammi visnaga** comes from a Mediterranean plant or a plant called Khellin. This plant has the active ingredient that is used in the drug Cromolyn sodium or Intal.

Use a couple of drops of Ammi oil in a diffuser and use once a day for a few weeks. It may take time for you to feel the results.

If you enjoy working and using essential oils, here is another combination that was created by Jeanne Rose and Victoria Edwards. Use this combination in a diffuser or vaporizer or you can add this blend in a base of flaxseed oil and rub on your chest just before you go to bed.

- 4 parts of Eucalyptus polybractea
- 1 part Hyssop cineol
- 1 part Inula graveolens
- 2 parts Basil eugenol
- 2 parts Lavender
- 2 parts Myrrh
- 3 parts Ammi visnaga
- 3 parts Chamomile, Roman
- 1 part Peppermint

This is quite a mixture of essential oils. But, mix them and put them in a brown dropper bottle and they will keep for a long time. They will give you relief when you need it the most.

Fennel seeds

Fennel seeds are also good for relieving asthma symptoms. Use it as a tea and get relief for asthma or other respiratory ailments.   Fennel contains rutin, vitamins, and minerals such as calcium and potassium.

Chapter 10: Foods to Eat When You Have Asthma

The best diet for the asthmatic is a vegetarian diet since it is this type of diet that will keep the asthmatic's body alkaline and free of mucus. Acids that are produced through various foods and activities will be neutralized quickly with a vegetarian diet. This can reduce or eliminate asthma symptoms or attacks.

There are many asthmatics that cannot follow a vegetarian diet and feel more comfortable eating meat. A well-balanced diet and eating specific highly alkaline foods can produce good results in reducing the effects of asthma.

Foods for reducing mucus

The foods that help asthma are those that thin down mucus. These are the foods that cause your nose to run. Some foods to add to your list are cinnamon, vinegar, pepper, garlic, onions, fish, tea, figs, grapes and fruits and vegetables that are high in vitamin C. Vitamin C helps to reduce inflammation.

Eating **apples** and drinking apple juice and fig juice will help you have fewer problems with colds and respiratory conditions. These fruits are alkaline food.

Eating **chili peppers** will cause watery secretions in the bronchioles thinning down the mucus and causing it to flow out. This helps in opening up the bronchioles so you can breathe easier.

Omega-3 fatty acids found in oils and fish are excellent to eat. These fatty acids help to reduce inflammation wherever it occurs in the body.

Using omega-3 and omega-6 oils are important when you have asthma. In fact, it is necessary even when you are not sick.

Foods, which are high in **vitamin C**, also help to reduce inflammation.

Foods or nutrients that promote your immune system also help to increase the level at which you will trigger an asthma attack. Use and rotate nutrients that increase immunity – **Echinacea, colostrums, and zinc**, acidophilus, beta-1,3glucan, coenzyme Q10, Selenium, glutathione, pycnogenol, superoxide dismutase (SOD),

Eat plenty of **citrus fruits**, bananas, grapes, whole grains, and green leafy vegetables. Also, eat more soups and liquid-like foods since they will reduce the thickness of mucus.

Eat plenty of vegetables since they are alkaline and help reduce the amount of acids in your body. Excess acid in your blood and in the lymph liquid that surrounds your cells can lead to asthma attacks.

In the morning, drink distilled water with the juice of **one lemon** without sugar, but you can add honey. During the day you can drink this drink or just drink plain water. Liquids help to move mucus build up in the bronchioles out of your body.

Lemon is acidic in the stomach, but when digested and used up in the cells they leave behind an alkaline residue that helps neutralize acids.

Drink rice dream, soymilk, or **almond milk** instead of milk, since milk is an acid food causes mucus. Raw **goats milk** is excellent and is a high alkaline food. Use raw goat milk or goat yogurt with acidophilus.

You can experiment with eating some of the more exotic grains such as amaranth, millet, quinoa, brown rice, and whole oats. But don't eat these for breakfast. Learn how to eat only fruits and fruit and vegetable juices only in the morning as outline in my Kindle book called, "**Secret Healthy Fruit Practices Revealed.**" Read the Kindle to find out about the natural body cycles that you can use to remove mucus from your body.

Avoid foods that create mucus – ice cream, sugar products, refined and processed foods, bread, milk, dairy products, and eggs.

The FDA has approved 1000's of food additives. Many of these spark allergic reactions and asthma attacks in many people. It is best to minimize the use of processed foods and move toward a more natural diet.

Avoid food products that have yellow dye #5, MSG and sulfides used to dry fruits. Look at the food labels and you will see that many foods have dyes, which you should avoid.

Eating sugar or an excess of sugar can bring on more asthma attacks.

Don't eat foods high in saturated fats, hydrogenated oils, safflower, or corn oils. Avoid eating lots of meat, margarine, and fried foods. If you like butter, use only natural butter and avoid margarine.

Cut back on meat. Eating excess meat is the foundation of many diseases including asthma. Meat is a highly acidic food. When too much meat is eaten, the liver, kidney, and intestines have too much protein and this weakens them. When you eat an excess of meat, too much ammonia is created, which the liver has to convert to urea and the body has to excrete it. But if the liver is filled with protein it cannot convert the ammonia over to urea.

Excess ammonia in the blood creates a condition called "alkalosis" an extremely toxic condition that weakens your immune system and your body. There can be different levels of alkalosis, so the less meat you eat the better your body function.

Sunflower Seeds

Sunflower seeds, high in protein, B-vitamins, and polyunsaturated oil are useful as a diuretic and as an expectorant for the bronchioles and lungs. Eat sunflowers seeds daily. It is best to buy them unsalted with shells. Sunflower seeds that are shelled have oil that gradually becomes rancid and toxic.

My daughter, a Nutritional Educator, who has suffered from asthma for most of her adult life talks about a diet she used to keep her Asthma under control.

"Basically I try to eat foods and drink fluids that will reduce inflammation and clear mucus. I stick to hot herbal teas, fresh vegetable juices, fish, salads, lightly steamed vegetables with squeezed lemon, and lots and lots of water.

Drinking herbal teas such as Mullein, Thyme or Green Tea will help break up the mucus, which is what we want to do. Green tea contains theophylline, which dilates the bronchial tubes. You can buy any of these teas or lung tea combinations at your local health food store.

Carrot juice is also good for breaking up mucus. I juice carrots in the morning and when I get home from work. I juice up one cup of organic carrot juice and add ½ - 1 cup of water to dilute it.

Fish is good to eat, in particular, Salmon, because it contains the Omega-3 essential fatty acids, which help reduce inflammation. Try to eat fish three times a week.

When buying your fish make sure it is not "Farmed." Farmed fish are not grown, treated, or fed properly. They are raised in small quarters and fed a pellet diet.

Buy fish caught in Alaska, because it is illegal to farm fish in that state. Fish from Alaska is caught in the deep ocean and is wild. The best fish is Alaskan Sockeye Salmon. Albacore White Tuna is also a good source of Omega-3's. If you do not like fish, take a good Omega-3 or a fish oil supplement daily.

One last thing is to drink water, lots of it. This is a simple thing to do but is often overlooked. Water will help clear your body of toxins, chemicals, and mucus. Keep a water bottle with you at all times and keep refilling it until you drink at least 8 – 12 glasses a day.

It's all about reducing inflammation, clearing the mucus and feeling good. Enjoy and happy eating!"

Footbath

Here is an herbal formula that you can use first thing in the morning or evening after your work.

Maurice Messegue, a famous herbalist, developed this formula during 1972.

Footbaths are soothing to use, but more importantly, herb nutrients and chemicals are easily absorbed through the bottom of your feet. Within minutes these nutrients are flowing in your bloodstream.

In your hot footbath, place equal amounts of herbs into the footbath. I usually mix the herbs first in a quart mason jar and shake to mix them up. Put 5 tablespoons of each herb into the jar.

Boil two cups of distilled water and then add 2-3 tablespoons of mixed herbs into the water and simmer for 15-20 minutes. Strain the mixture and when the bath is hot, put the liquid herbs into the bath. Cut the garlic into large pieces and put them straight into the footbath.

- One cut head of garlic

- Corn poppy

- Lavender

- Parsley

- Ground ivy

- Sage

- Thyme

If you are missing one herb, don't worry about it. It is better to do a footbath with the herbs that you can get than to not do the footbath.

Place your feet into the footbath with herbs and garlic. Do this for 15 – 20 minutes every day.

If you don't see results in 4 –5 days don't give up. I usually use a footbath for 20- 30 days and then rest. Then, later in the year, I do it again just for blood circulation and good health.

Some people respond very well to the footbath, while others simply get some relief. The herbs listed here for asthma are not just for asthma but have many other health benefits.

Ginkgo Biloba Extract

Ginkgo is a well-known herb that helps to increase blood circulation throughout the body. For asthmatics, it's critical to keep the capillaries open that pick up oxygen from the tiny sacs called "alveoli" that are in the lungs. If these get plugged up from free radical damage, you will experience an asthma attack. Using Ginkgo will help prevent the free radical damage of these capillaries.

Ginkgo has another important action in that it blocks the chemical "platelet activating factor", PAF. PAF is called into action by the immune system to release mucus as a result of some irritating conditions. Sometimes PAF overreacts and releases too much mucus and this is where using ginkgo can help block PAF.

If you have asthma, this overreaction can lead to a strong asthma attack. Ginkgo blocks PAF so your body can't overreact and so your asthma attacks are less frequent and less severe.

Take Ginkgo long term by using an extract. Use a dose of 80 – 160 milligrams spread out into three parts.

Green Drink

A green drink is a powerful drink that can help detoxify your colon and your blood. This drink keeps your colon and your whole body working better and longer by preventing toxic gases from forming in the colon and forcing toxins into your blood.

There are many types of green drinks that are prepared with powders. But the green drink that I like is made using only liquid chlorophyll.

Chlorophyll has many benefits. It is capable of neutralizing substances that cause cell mutations and strengthens the cell walls of the small intestine and colon. It has an exceptional deodorizing effect on your body and on the stools you have during a bowel movement.

I drink my green drink the first thing in the morning on an empty stomach. This helps to activate your colon and stimulate it to have a bowel movement.

Here's how I prepare my green drink.

Add 1-2 oz of pure liquid chlorophyll into an empty glass (you may want to start with a tablespoon or two until you get used to the taste)

- Squeeze the juice of one lemon into the glass

- Fill the glass with 8 oz of distilled water

- Drink the combination completely

I add lemon juice to the chlorophyll because chlorophyll has a dull and blank taste that I don't like. With lemon, it's a drink that I enjoy taking every morning.

If you have other health issues you want to work on, you can add other nutrients or liquids to this green drink. You can add a few drops of a product called Oxygen Elements Plus, which also is good for constipation and helps to detoxify your colon even more. You can add Alkalife, an alkaline water booster, which adds minerals to your drink and helps neutralize body acids.

From the clients that I have worked with, I have found that this chlorophyll drink helps them get better blood test results. Their blood is a little thinner. They carry more oxygen into the cells. Their blood cell count goes up.

Use this drink and you will keep drinking it every morning just like I do, especially if you like lemon juice.

Chapter 11: Herbs The Reduce Asthma Attacks

Herbs that are useful in asthma are those that have expectorant and anti-inflammatory properties. The herbs with expectorant properties help to change the quantity and quality of the mucus in the bronchioles and lungs. Then, they expel the mucus by making you cough or by way of the lymph system.

Here are some herbs that help eliminate mucus from the lungs and bronchioles. Look for them in herbal mixtures:

Lobelia – extract can be used during an asthma attack. It is a bronchial muscle relaxant. Use it by putting a few drops into water and drinking it.

Licorice – one of most often used herbs in Chinese herbalism, which acts as a tonic for the whole body. It also has specific action as an expectorant for the lungs and a cough suppressant. It has anti-allergy action like cortisone but not as strong.

Grindella

This herb is found in the United States and is called the gum plant. It is used for arthritis, to cleanse the kidney, to slow the heartbeat, and for asthma as an expectorant.

Use this herb with care since a small dose can irritate the kidneys and large doses can be poisonous. Just follow the instructions on the product label.

Stinging nettles

Stinging nettles have anti-inflammatory effects and are useful in reducing the inflammation in the bronchial tubes. It may also have some anti-histamine activity.

Use stinging nettles as a tea and drink 1-2 cups or as needed. Add a heaping tablespoon of this herb into 2 cups of hot distilled water and let simmer for 10 minutes.

Yerba Santa

This herb is an excellent expectorant and is used when you have a lot of mucus. Use it as a tea for asthma, mucus, throat and bronchial irritations.

As with most herbal teas or herbal capsules, it is best that pregnant women not use them unless they have been tested as ok for pregnancies.

Here's a tea or infusion that you can make to get asthma relief.

- 1 part garden thyme
- 1 part wild thyme
- 1 part rosemary
- 1 part vervain

In making a tea or infusion, put a tablespoon of herbal mixture into 2 cups of hot distilled water and let sit for 10 –15 minutes. Then strain, let cool a little more and drink. You may want to add a slight amount of honey if the taste is too strong.

Chinese herbs and formulas

Here's a tea that is used by Chinese to alleviate asthma. Mix equal parts of the following herbs and make a tea and drink daily.

Ling Zhi or Reishi Mushroom

- Peppermint
- Basil

Another Chinese remedy calls for roasting an orange with a chopstick to hold it. Then, eat only the inside of the orange, each day for seven days.

Daniel B. Mowrey, Ph. D. in his book, The Scientific

Validation of Herbal Medicine gives a useful formula for asthma. Here are the herbs to mix or to find already mixed.

- Pleurisy root
- Wild cherry bark
- Slippery elm bark
- Plantain

- Mullein leaves
- Chickweed
- Horehound
- Licorice root
- Kelp
- Cayenne
- Saw Palmetto

Herbs to use as teas

Use any of the following herbs individually or mix 2-3 of them to make a tea:

Mullein, eucalyptus, watercress, saw palmetto, burdock root, chamomile, elecampane root, flaxseeds, ground ivy horseradish, lungwort, or parsley.

Ayurveda Herbs

Here is a lung formula containing India herbs that have a strengthening action on the lungs, bronchioles and improves your immune system.

This formula is easily available on the Internet under the name "Lung Formula" and contains the following herbs:

- Licorice root
- Cane Sugar
- Pippali fruit

- Elecampane root
- Vasaka leaf
- Amalaki fruit
- Bibhitaki fruit
- Haritaki fruit
- Tulsi leaf
- Cardamom seed
- Talisa leaf
- Cinnamon bark

Here's where you can get this Lung Formula:
Lung Formula

Andrew Weil, M.D., in his book **Spontaneous Healing, 1995**, talks about a patient with a difficult case of asthma. The person was taking multiple drugs, using inhalers, eating a strict diet, using vitamins, and testing alternative methods without improvement. It was only until he sought out an Ayurvedic practitioner that he finally started to improve.

Here's what Andrew Weil recommends for tough asthma cases,

"Bronchial asthma is not one disease but several. Some forms respond more easily to treatment than others. Allopathic measures are toxic and addictive, yet it is often impossible to do without them. The potential for spontaneous healing of asthma is significant, especially with major lifestyle change or application of alternative medical methods. The Ayurvedic approach, with its emphasis on the right diet for each person and its wealth of medicinal plants upon which to draw, might be worth exploring if you have a stubborn, chronic disease that conventional medicine cannot cure."

Honey

Using honey for asthma and other respiratory illness makes sense since honey has an antibacterial effect. Honey draws out the moisture from bacteria and kills them dead.

Use honey that is unfiltered, unheated, and dark. This type of honey contains more levulose, a type of sugar molecule that is absorbed into the blood slowly and does not cause the blood sugar to rise too fast.

Here is a recipe that has been used by many people and you can use when you have to deal with asthma every day. It reduces inflammation and continual coughing.

Cut up 3-5 slices of onions

Cut up a clove of garlic

Place this in 16 oz of Irish moss jelly and simmer for 30 minutes. After it cools add 4 – 5 ounces of local organic raw honey. Mix in well and, Take one teaspoon every other hour and one teaspoon of pure honey every alternate hour.

Another way of using honey, garlic, and onions is to soak slices of onions and garlic in honey overnight. The next day, stir the mixture to spread the onion and garlic juices into the honey.

Or, If you have a juicer or a garlic press you can press out the onion and garlic juice and let this sit overnight in some honey.

The next day, take this mixture 3 – 4 times during the day.

Using **eucalyptus honey** makes this remedy even more powerful since eucalyptus leaves have a healing effect for asthma and help to break down mucus that forms in the bronchioles.

Juices

A combination of two ounces each of **carrots, onions, and parsley juice** provides a drink that helps relax the bronchial muscles and prevent spasms. Take this drink twice a day.

Another juice, which is quite helpful in asthma, is a combination of **carrot, celery, and endive**. Endive is one of the richest sources of vitamin A in a vegetable.

This juice combination is highly alkaline and will neutralize a lot of body acid.

Use twice as much carrot juice in these juice combinations.

Here are other juice combinations you can use:

- Carrot, celery
- Carrot, radish
- Carrot, celery, radish

Grapefruit   juice   with   Aloe   Vera

Here is a natural remedy that comes from Puerto Rico. Take Fresh grapefruit juice and combine it with fresh, peeled, finely chopped aloe vera. Then drink this combination. Start with 1 glass per day and work up to 2 glasses per day.

Another way you can try this drink if fresh aloe vera is not available is to use whole leaf organic aloe vera. Here is where you can get it already made.

Grapefruit Whole Leaf Aloe Vera Juice

Or, you can make your own by adding 2 oz of aloe vera to the 6 oz grapefruit and then add more aloe as you get used to the taste. You may have to start with less aloe vera if you like.

Another way to use this combination is to use aloe vera capsules and drink them with 6 – 8 oz of grapefruit juice.

Aloe Vera has anti-inflammatory properties and can heal open wounds by promoting cell regeneration. Grapefruit contains vitamin C and plenty of bioflavonoids that can prevent tissue damage from free radicals.

Do not use this drink after taking drugs, since grapefruit juice increases the effects of drugs.

Manganese

Manganese is called the "love element" because people who lack it shows signs of meanness, vindictiveness, lacking love, and are anti-social. It is found in the linings of the brain, in the nerves, in the lining of the heart, and in the blood. It helps carry oxygen from the lungs to the cells.

Manganese strengthens the lining of the bronchioles and makes them more elastic.

Manganese works with certain enzymes to help cells use fat, protein, and carbohydrate. It helps protect the cells from free radical damage.

There are indications that people with asthma are low in manganese. Your diet should include those foods that are high in manganese.

Peas, beans, blueberries, nuts – Missouri black walnuts, almonds, pecans - and seeds – sesame -, buckwheat, cardamon, marjoram, rye bread, pumpernickel bread, and steel cut oats, apples, apricots, black-eyed peas, celery, parsley, watercress, wheat bran, wheat germ, whole grains, avocados, and cantaloupes.

Pineapple is another source high in manganese. It also is high in vitamins A and C.

Taking electrolyte manganese liquid will also supply you with ionic manganese that is ready to use by your body. Here where you can get liquid manganese:

Electrolyte Manganese

MSM, MethylSulfonylMethane

MSM is organic sulfur. It is now widely available in capsule, pill, or powder form and in different purity grades.

In their book, MSM The Definitive Guide, 2003, Stanley W. Jacob, M.D., FL.A.C.S., and Jeremy Appleton, N. D., talk about an individual that came to their clinic with asthma,

"AA had been hospitalized for seven months (multiple admissions) for asthma. She experienced frequent attacks, beginning with wheezing, coughing, and shortness of breath: this was followed by respiratory distress. Her therapy had included antihistaminic agents, theophylline, and corticosteroids.

We administered oral MSM, starting with a ¼ teaspoon of powder (approximately 1 gram) twice daily. We gradually increased her dosage to 8 grams per day. She remains on this dosage at the time of this writing and has not required hospitalization for three years."

MSM is an anti-inflammatory and is used to reduce arthritic pain. But it is useful in reducing inflammation in any part of the body including inflammation of the bronchioles.

In my constipation book, I recommend it as a method of relieving constipation. As you increase the amount of MSM you take it will get your bowels moving. I found for me around 8 – 10 gram per day, spread over the day, is enough to give me 4 bowel movements per day.

MSM helps the body keep its acid-alkaline balance. It also helps in the creation and regeneration of the body's tissues. MSM is found in every body cell and helps to keep the cells soft so nutrients can easily go into the cell and waste can easily come out of the cell. This easy movement of chemicals, in and out of the cell, helps the body recover from illness quicker and helps to make your body healthier.

Here's how to use MSM:

During the first week: Take 3 grams or 1 gram with each meal

During the second week: Take 4 – 6 grams or 2 grams per meal

During the third week: Take 8 – 12 grams or 4 grams per meal

During the fourth week: Take 16 – 24 grams or 5 or more grams per meal.

You can reduce the amount of MSM you take when you are seeing too many bowel movements.

Mullein Tea

Mullein tea has been found to be useful in asthma if taken every day. It is slow to show results but continual use will provide lasting results in asthma relief.

Make a tea out of dried or fresh leaves. Simmer for 10 – 15 for a stronger tea.

Oxygen

When you have an asthma attack, your body is struggling for oxygen. Here are some things that you can add to your diet that can bring in more oxygen into your body cells.

Vitamin E – use 400 IU

Fish oil – take as directed on the bottle

Digestive enzymes with HCl – use 1-2 capsules per meal

Relaxation

People have lessened their asthma attacks by learning self-hypnosis and relaxation. By learning yoga breathing exercises you can improve your asthma and have fewer attacks.

In the book, High-Speed Healing, 1991, by Prevention Editors, they report that Dr. Schenkel says, "Short of medication, what I often recommend for asthma is relaxation. What happens with asthma if you're hungry for air so you panic and the panic tends to make asthma worse.

Simply relaxing the way you usually relax is one of the best treatments you can give yourself — and relaxation can help soothe an asthma attack in about 15 to 20 minutes."

Dr. Bach has developed a blend of flower remedies that help you relax when you have anxiety as when you feel an asthma attack coming. He has developed an array of flower remedies that help in emotional and psychological problems.

The flower remedy to use for asthma is found under the names:

- Calming Essence,
- Rescue Remedy
- Five-Flower Formula
- Emergency Stress Relief Formula

Here's how to use it. Place 4 drops under the tongue and hold there for a minute so that the flower nutrients are absorbed into the blood. You can also add four drops into a glass of distilled water and sip it slowly.

The intent of using these flower remedies is to calm you when you feel anxious or to calm you when you feel an asthma attack looming.

Pressure Points

Here are a couple of spots that you can press to prevent an asthma attack or to lessen one if you are having one.

Press the points on both sides of your body just below the collar and two-three inches away from the center of the collarbone for 2 minutes. Hang your head down and breath slowly and deeply as you press.

Vitamins and Minerals

Vitamin C is important in reducing asthma attacks. It is able to stop bronchial constriction and reduce histamine production and release. It also helps to lower histamine levels, after histamine is released into the blood. So take between 2000 mg to 4000 mg per day. Spread them out to 3 times per day with each meal. Use Ester C if other Vitamin C supplements give you stomach problems.

If you have diarrhea when taking vitamin C, just back off on the amount you are taking, until you have no more diarrhea.

Taking **antioxidant** nutrients is also good since they help to protect from free radical damage and irritation. Take 400 IU of vitamin E and 10,000 IU of beta-carotene.

Take a supplement of **magnesium** or get it in foods such as whole grains, or seafood. Use around 400 mg of magnesium aspartate twice a day.

Vitamin B12 has been found to be essential in relieving childhood asthma. In clinical trails injections of 1000 ug of B12 created improvement in patients with asthma. B12 is most helpful in people with sulfite sensitivities. Taking B12 capsules would be helpful prior to any meal.

Vitamin B6 has also been found to reduce the frequency and severity of asthma attacks and wheezing. By taking the B100's you can get all of the B vitamins. Take 50 milligrams two times a day.

Quercetin is a flavonoid. A flavonoid is a chemical in fruits and flowers that give them their color. Quercetin has a high activity against asthma and acts somewhat similar to the drug Cromolyn. What quercetin does is block the release of histamine from "mast cells." When it does this, it substantially reduces the irritation and inflammation reaction to allergens.

Also, quercetin blocks another inflammatory substance that is released by the "mast cells" called leukotriene. This substance is a thousand times more powerful and harmful than histamine.

Since the body does not readily absorb quercetin, it is best to take it with bromelain to improve its absorption. Here's where to get this combination:

- Quercetin Bromelain
- Quercetin twice a day at 300mg
- N-acetylcysteine twice a day at 500 mg

Chapter 12: Summary and Final Comments

There are many causes of asthma and each person can have different asthma attack triggers. So, each person may need to use a different medical approach and different natural remedy.

Using drugs to control your asthma makes sense when you first discover that you have asthma provided your asthma is life-threatening. Once you have your prescriptions and your doctor's instructions, you should consider looking at or experimenting with natural remedies to control or even eliminate your asthma, since drugs are not a cure.

No matter what type of drug or inhaler you are using, they all have their side effects. The longer you use drugs or an inhaler, the less effective they will be and the more likely you will see side effects.

You should use natural remedies when you are having an asthma attack or when asthma is under control. With so many natural remedies that I have given you, you may not know where to start. There are four areas you need to concentrate on:

- Reduce mucus
- Reduce inflammation
- Reduce emotional and stressful situation

- Improve immune system

Reduce Mucus

By using various herbs you can control and remove mucus from your bronchioles. Test various herbs or herbal combinations to determine which work best for you.

Drink carrot and celery juice and drink plenty of water daily to help dilute and move mucus out of your body.

Reduce Inflammation

There are quite a few different nutrients that can help you reduce inflammation. You should consider using more than one at a time. Start with these and then experiment with the others.

Add omega-3 to your diet by using flaxseed oil or fish oil Use MSM supplements.

- Take vitamin C supplement
- Systemic enzymes, try Vitalzyme
- Digestive enzymes

Reduce Emotional and Stressful Situation

Reducing stress in your life is a difficult area to deal with since some situations in your life are strongly anchored, like your job, your family, your friends, or marital situation. But if these areas are causing your stress and you frequently have asthma attacks, then you have to decide which is more important for you, your job or your health.

If your job is deteriorating your health, then start looking for a way out. This may require you to look for another job or to go back to school to get training for something you might like to do.

Just take action and start changing your life. By doing nothing, you will stay in the same place. So take even small steps to change your life for the good.

Improve Immune System

Improving your immune system is accomplished through diet, by taking nutritional supplements, by reducing stress, and eliminating those conditions that overwork your body.

The fewer things your immune system has to react to and get under control, the stronger it is to take care of a health crisis when it occurs. When your immune system has to deal with toxins in your colon and throughout your body, then it is weakened and not able to neutralize pollen or pollution you inhale from the air.

When your immune system is busy trying to neutralize acids from the food you eat daily, it may not have time to react properly to the stress from your job. The result can be bronchiole spasms that lead to an asthma attack.

Final Words

First, Start using the various natural remedies to help elevate your immune system and to strengthen your internal organs. Change your diet as recommended so that you make your body more alkaline. Eat the type of foods that do not create mucus – more raw vegetables and fruits and their juices. Stay away from foods that create mucus – excessive meat, milk, wheat, bread, white flour products, packaged foods, and sugary products.

Take action to change the stressful areas of your life. Add more relaxations, physical and yoga exercise to your lifestyle. And, it can just be walking around the block every day.

Start working with your doctor, as you use more natural remedies, to reduce your medication. This should be your primary goal to slowly move off medication. Drugs or other types of medication should be used short term and not long term. Using drugs long term can be detrimental to your health and intensify your asthma attacks.

Dosages to take

Here is a guideline on the dosages of various herbal products or supplements that you should use if you have children or teens:

- Ages 2 – 5 years use ¼ the adult dose
- Ages 6 – 12 years use ½ the adult dose
- Ages 13 – 17 years use ¾ the adult dose

When giving children natural remedies, use common sense in the amounts you give. If a child has a big body structure, then they will require a little bit more and if a child is small they will require less.

In making eating habits and lifestyle changes and taking more nutrients and supplements, start out slow and easy so that you don't overwhelm yourself with changes. Do one small step at a time. When you do this then the changes will more likely stick, then if you tried to do a whole bunch of things right away.

Good luck and good health to you.

If you have any questions, feel free to email me at: rudysilva@comcast.net
And don't forget to visit my other site for more health information.

Rudy Silva, Natural Nutritionist

Constipation health remedies

Acid Reflux information

Hair loss remedies

Clear Your Acne

Arthritis Pain relief

Hemorrhoid Information

Stop Constipation

Asthma Relief

About The Author

Rudy Silva is a Natural Nutritionist and a graduated from the Bauer's College of Nutrition, which is located in San Rafael,

California. He also has a degree in Physics from San Jose University.

Rudy has written over 200 natural remedy health articles that appear throughout the Internet. He has helped many clients with their nutritional health issues.

He writes a weekly newsletter called "Natural Remedies Thatwork.com." This newsletter details various ways you can deal with poor health. Natural remedies are discussed, such as using vitamins, minerals, food, herbs, special nutritional formulations, and certain nutritional supplements to bring you back to normal health.

You can sign up for his newsletter here and receive a special report call, "creating long-term acceptable health."http://www.natural-remedies-thatwork.com.

Here are several e-books that he has written in the natural remedy field.

1. Seven Day Colon and Blood Cleansing Diet – this e-book gives a step by step method of doing a colon and blood cleanse using fruits, vegetables, and their juices.

2. Constipation Natural Cures – this is a comprehensive e-book on all aspects of constipation and colon health. In this e-book, you will find all the information you need on how your colon really works and what you need to do to get rid of constipation.

3. Acne Natural Treatments – This e-book outlines internal and external processes to use to stop the progression of facial acne. Natural remedies are given so that you can minimize the growth of pimples. You also are given a facial technique with various creams so that you can eliminate the external facial blemishes.

4. Hemorrhoid Natural Remedies - A variety of different remedies and techniques are outlined and given so that you can eliminate your hemorrhoids. Some remedies are provided from feedback given by clients.

5. Asthma Remedies – In this e-book, my daughter and I worked together to create a process that will help you minimize and even eliminated asthma using natural remedies. She has had asthma for many years and has discovered what diet she had to follow to prevent asthma attacks. This diet is provided with a variety of the most effective natural remedies that work on asthma and asthma attacks.

6. Essential Fatty Acids Explained – in this e-book, you will discover how essential fatty acids – omega-3 and omega-6 – work in your body. You will learn what diseases are created when you are deficient in essential fatty acids. Knowing this information will help you avoid these diseases and help you live a longer productive and pleasurable life.

7 Acid Reflux and Heartburn Diet – Gain a full understanding of what acid reflux is. Using this information, you will be able to see why the diet given really works. You will discover the natural remedies that you need to use to stabilize your stomach and to rejuvenate the tissue damage done in your stomach acid and in your esophagus.

"Hey don't forget to leave a review for this e-booklet on the Amazon website next to my booklet. It will be sincerely appreciated."

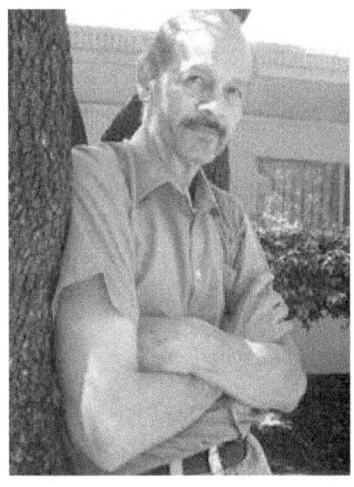

"To Your Good Health and Long Strong Life"

Rudy S. Silva, Natural Nutritionist